Ketogenic Diet for Beginners

The Complete Low-Carb Guide for Optimal Weight Loss

Charles Kelso

Contents

Introduction to the Ketogenic Diet 1

  Keto Dieting in a Nutshell 1

  Ketosis is a Game Changing Revelation 2

    Ketosis Leads to Natural Weight Loss 2

    Low Carb Foods Keep your Appetite Under Control 3

    Ketones Promote Better Mental Focus 3

    You'll Have Much More Energy 4

    It Helps Fight Type II Diabetes 4

    Boosts Your HDL Cholesterol 5

  Reading and Understanding Food Labels 5

    Carbohydrates 6

    Ingredients 6

Chapter 1 8

  Macros and the Ketogenic Diet 9

  Becoming Keto-Adaptive 9

  Checking Your Ketone Levels 10

    Urine Testing 10

    Breath Testing 11

    Blood Testing 11

Chapter 2 12

  Low-Carb Foods 12

  Fats and Oils 13

  Protein-Based Foods 14

  Vegetables and Fruits 16

Dairy Products 17

Nuts and Seeds 19

  Making Flours Using Nuts and Seeds.............................20

Beverages..20

  Important Hydration Note..21

Spices and Cooking in a Keto-Friendly Way.....................22

Condiments and Sauces...23

Sweeteners 25

  Sugar Addiction..26

Finding Hidden Carbs 27

Foods That You Should Avoid 29

Chapter 3 31

  They Are Usually Very Small 31

  They Can Be Sweet or Savory...32

  They Should Be Loaded with Healthy Fat.........................32

  Fat Bombs Are Refrigerated 32

  They Usually Contain Nuts and Seeds 32

Three Easy Steps to Make Your Own Fat Bombs 33

  Step 1..34

  Step 2..34

  Step 3..34

Four Amazing Fat Bomb Recipes! 36

Chapter 4 42

Carbohydrates 42

Protein...43

Fats 44

Calculating Macros 44

Macro Calculators 46

Chapter 5 47

The Four Types of Exercise That Best Compliment the Ketogenic Diet..47

Aerobic Exercise 48

Anaerobic Exercise 48

Flexibility Exercises...48

Stability Exercises 48

How to Target Ketogenic Dieting to Our Exercise 49

Ketogenic Adaptation 49

Why Exercise is Beneficial for Ketosis 49

Best Exercise for Keto Dieters 50

Chapter 6 51

Support Makes the Journey Easier......................................51

Focus on Positives Rather Than Negatives.........................51

Deal with Setbacks Immediately 52

Start Your Day on a Positive Note 52

Continuously Educate Yourself About Health 53

Final Thoughts 54

Four-Week 57

Ketogenic 57

Meal 57

Plan 57

Meal Plan Introduction 59

Week 1 60

Week 2 62

Week 3 64

Week 4 66

Recipes 69

Get an Audio Book for FREE! 116

One Last Thing... Did You Enjoy the Book? 117

Get an Audio Book for FREE!

Don't have an Audible account?

Sign up and get "Ketogenic Diet for beginners" audio book for FREE!

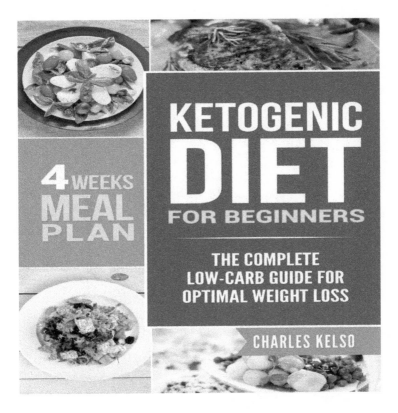

http://bit.ly/kelso-keto-diet

Introduction to the Ketogenic Diet

When people first started hearing about this new diet where they can eat foods that are higher in fat, it quickly became the chatter of the entire world. Many people are still reluctant to believe that a diet that's high in fatty foods could be healthy. One of the first questions that people ask is, *"What makes the ketogenic diet so good?"*

Before we get into the benefits associated with the ketogenic diet, let's take a closer look at what it is.

Keto Dieting in a Nutshell

The goal of the keto diet is to get your body to fall into a metabolic state known as ketosis. To accomplish that end, we focus on foods that are low in carbs but high in fat.

Ketosis is the metabolic state that the body falls into when it runs out of glycogen reserves. Think about it like this: The body stores fat so that it has an energy reserve to fall back on, so the trick is to get the body to burn these fats. That will only happen when the body runs out of glycogen (sugars/carbs) because it searches for another fuel source. When that happens, the liver will start to break down fat and process it. In that instance, ketones become the body's main source of fuel.

We'll be digging deeper into this process throughout the course of this book. For now, here is ketosis in a nutshell:

High fat + low carbs = body burns fat as fuel (Ketosis)

High carbs = body burns glycogen and stores fat (weight gain)

Ketosis is a Game Changing Revelation

You can create some of the most amazing recipes under the ketogenic diet—recipes that allow you to add delicious oils and butter to your meals. In fact, you will have to add them in a lot of cases just to reach the targeted amount of fat.

Keto dieting is more of a lifestyle than an actual diet. It has effectively changed the lives of so many people. This book will lay out a program that shows you how to transform your body into a fat burning machine!

Most diets do well in helping you shed weight, at least in the beginning. But for many, they are just too strict, so it's easy to fall off the wagon. Once you fall off, your metabolic rate is so out of sync that it leads to even more weight gain than before, leading to depression and binge eating.

That's why ketosis is so beneficial. It relies on a natural chemistry in your body to promote weight loss. Plus, the body is more efficient when it uses ketones as a source of fuel.

With that in mind, let's look at some of the main benefits of the ketogenic diet.

Ketosis Leads to Natural Weight Loss

Most of you are reading this book with this sole benefit in mind, so it's the best place to start. When fat becomes the primary source of energy, your body will stop storing fat. Instead, it burns it as energy.

The process looks something like this:

You stop consuming glucose. After a short period of time, the body will run out of glycogen.

Introduction to the Ketogenic Diet

The body enters ketosis as soon as it runs out of glycogen. This causes your blood sugar and insulin to drop.

Fat cells start to release water that they have been storing. This in itself leads to a great deal of weight loss. It's the reason why people drop a lot of weight very quickly.

Once that water is lost, the fat cells become small enough to enter into the bloodstream where the liver can then convert them into ketones. This process will continue as you progress through the keto journey!

Low Carb Foods Keep your Appetite Under Control

When your diet isn't heavy in carbs, you will find that your appetite is not as great as it once was. You'll stay full for longer periods of time without experiencing cravings. The Achilles's Heel of all diets is random cravings that cause us to crave unhealthy foods like donuts and other sugary treats.

In fact, a lot of people who try the keto diet are surprised at how little they crave food. When you're not constantly looking for things to eat, you'll find that it's much easier to follow through with a dieting plan.

Ketones Promote Better Mental Focus

The problem with carbs as a primary energy source is that they cause rapid spikes and dips in your blood sugar levels. When our energy source is not a constant, it's much more difficult for the mind to stay focused for longer periods of time. The mind craves consistency.

When in ketosis, the brain will pull from those ketones as a primary source of fuel. Since it's a much more consistent fuel source, it means that you'll be able to focus for longer periods of time. Your mind will be sharp, rather than cloudy.

It's difficult to explain the feeling because you probably don't even realize that your mind is not operating at 100 percent. You're used to being bogged down by rapidly shifting blood sugar levels, but once you get into ketosis, you will start to notice the difference.

You'll Have Much More Energy

Your body is only able to store a specific amount of glycogen. That's why you get hungry all throughout the day when consuming a lot of carbs. It also means that you will have to constantly refuel in order to maintain enough energy to operate efficiently.

Since your body can store more fat, it becomes a fuel source that will never run out. That's also why you have fewer cravings on the ketosis diet. This also means that you will have much more energy throughout the day.

Imagine not feeling the afternoon drain that is common in so many people.

It Helps Fight Type II Diabetes

Those who suffer from Type II diabetes are dealing with increased production of insulin. Since the keto diet removes sugars completely from your diet, it serves as a natural counter to Type II diabetes. There have been numerous studies that have shown the keto diet to reduce key factors that relate to Type II diabetes.

So if you are suffering from this terrible disease, then you have found the perfect dieting plan to fight back!

Introduction to the Ketogenic Diet

Boosts Your HDL Cholesterol

Most people panic as soon as they hear the words "high cholesterol" in the same sentence but there are actually two types of cholesterol–HDL and LDL.

HDL is a beneficial cholesterol that moves cholesterol directly to the liver where it can either be reused or excreted.

LDL is a bad cholesterol that moves cholesterol away from the liver and into the body.

When your body is in ketosis, HDL cholesterol will increase while triglycerides decrease. The ratio of triglycerides-to-HDL is actually a determining factor in an individual's risk of heart disease. A higher ratio means that you have a greater risk of heart disease.

Reading and Understanding Food Labels

A lot of the battle in taking the keto journey is to learn to read labels effectively. This is not as easy as some people seem to think. Some companies are really good at hiding carbs behind fancy labels or using super small serving sizes. Here are some of the important parts of the label. Pay close attention to these.

Serving size: This is important because some companies use small serving sizes to hide the amount of carbs in their food. Be sure to pay close attention to this.

Total calories: While counting calories is not the most important part of the ketogenic diet, you still have to make sure that you remain at a calorie deficit. So this information is helpful.

Fats: The amount of fat is not really an issue, but the type of fat is very important. Stay away from trans-fat when possible.

Carbohydrates

There are several categories of carbs on a food label. It's important to understand each one. We are trying to aim for a low blood sugar impact.

Total carbohydrates: Always start by looking at the total grams of carbs. If it's really high, then put that food right back onto the shelf! Even if the carbs are from a "healthy source," they're going to cause our blood glucose to spike.

Fiber: This is a healthy type of carb that can actually be subtracted from "total carbs" to come up with a figure known as "net carbs." When dealing with ketosis, we only care about net carbs. Fiber does not raise our blood glucose level.

Sugars and sugar alcohol: Both are huge red flags. Avoid them at all costs. Products can be labeled as "sugar free" but still contain sugar alcohols. Some of them will actually spike your blood sugar levels, so it's a good idea to avoid them altogether. Please note that erythritol is a safe sugar alcohol.

Protein: It's important that we consume enough protein while on the keto diet since our body will be dependent on it. Protein also regulates our appetite. However, too much protein can actually throw us out of ketosis. This is why macros are so important.

Ingredients

There are certain ingredients that you need to be weary of when on the keto diet. Let's look at a few that you need to be on the lookout for because they have an impact on your blood sugar levels.

Refined and processed carbs: These are sugars, refined grains, and other things. Sugar can go by a lot of different aliases, including the infamous "high fructose corn syrup." "Evaporated cane juice" is another fancy name for sugar. There are also refined flours that you need to be on the lookout for.

Sugar alcohols: Make sure that there are no sugar alcohols on the ingredient list. There are times when companies do not have to place these under carbohydrates. But they always have to place them in the ingredient list.

I am going to be telling you to read labels throughout this book because it's important to maintaining ketosis.

Chapter 1
An In-Depth Look at the Ketogenic Diet

More people are starting to follow the ketogenic diet because of the amazing benefits that accompany it. For those of you who might still be a bit skeptical, let's take a deeper look at how it all works. What is it that makes this dieting plan such an amazing weight-loss tool?

As we saw in the introduction, the most basic fact about the ketogenic diet is that it gets the body to start burning fats as fuel, rather than relying on carbohydrates. The goal is to keep your carbohydrate intake low enough so that the body starts producing ketones. In short, the body wants to use carbohydrates as fuel, so if you do not remove them, then it's always going to use them. It will then store fat. However, removing carbohydrates forces the body to use fat as fuel rather than storing it. Think of fat as high-octane gasoline. When it's burned, the body's metabolism is given a significant boost and you will have a higher energy level.

If burning fat is so wonderful, then why doesn't the body do it all of the time? Our biology is centered around survival in an environment where we are forced to hunt for food on a daily basis. The problem is that society has outgrown our biology. Food is readily available, so the body storing fat as a way to prepare for long periods of time without food is detrimental since food is so convenient now.

In short, the body burns short term energy first and stores the best for when we need it most. The ketogenic diet forces the body to burn that high octane fuel now.

Macros and the Ketogenic Diet

Since the ketogenic diet is creating a biological reaction in your body, it's important that you carefully monitor your food intake. We use macros to keep track of whether certain recipes are okay when following this diet. Don't worry though. There are a number of different tools and I'm going to dedicate an entire chapter to macros later.

For now, I just want you to understand how it works. A keto macro is broken down into three categories: fat, protein, and carbs. Fat should be high, protein moderate, and carbs should be kept low.

By this point, you understand that the idea is to consume foods that are high in fat and low in carbs, but protein is where a lot of people drop the ball. Eating too much protein can actually have a detrimental effect on ketosis.

That means it's important to only consume a moderate amount of protein. The body will start to break down protein instead of fat, leading to the same problems that occur when your diet contains too many carbs.

Watching your protein consumption is just as important as watching your carb intake.

Macros will also vary from person-to-person, so you will need access to a macro calculator.

Becoming Keto-Adaptive

Ketosis is one of the most natural functions of the body. The process involves starving the body of carbs in order to condition it to burn fat as fuel.

When training your body to adapt to ketosis, it is going to put you through a tough time. Your body will fight it at first, and your metabolism might actually slow down for a few days, leading to a lack of energy. However, if you stick with it then your body will start to prefer burning fat.

In short, becoming keto-adaptive transforms your body into a fat burning machine.

It's also important that you drink enough water during this time.

Checking Your Ketone Levels

While it's certainly not absolutely necessary, it's still good practice to check your ketone levels frequently. It's the only way that you can know for sure whether or not you have entered ketosis. With that said, as long as you follow your macros diligently, you'll be okay. I do highly recommend that you check your ketone levels at least once per month, though.

When your body starts producing ketones, they spill over into the blood stream, urine, and even your breath. That makes it possible to test for them in all of those areas. There are several home testing methods available:

Urine Testing

Urine strips are used for testing ketone levels and can be bought at your local drugstore. The downside is that they are not always 100% reliable. As your body becomes more efficient at using ketones, your urine will contain fewer of them.

There are other factors that can affect the readings as well, such as hydration levels.

An In-Depth Look at the Ketogenic Diet

Breath Testing

When your body produces ketones, another compound called acetone will show up in your breath. You can test for this using a breath meter. The benefit of breath testing is that once you invest in the initial cost, there are no further expenses. But this is not the most reliable method, so it should not be the only method of testing you use.

Blood Testing

This is by far the most effective method of testing your ketone levels. By using a blood glucose meter, you can check your ketone levels with precise accuracy. This is also the most expensive and invasive method, so you should use it sparingly.

For the best results, you will want to provide your body with optimal nutrition based on the macro that fits your lifestyle. Then mix in the different testing methods to be sure your body is responding in the desired way.

Chapter 2
Foods to Get You Into Ketosis

Dieting is quite a complicated word because there are just so many different variations in the world. The most difficult part of any diet is knowing exactly what foods to eat and making sure you avoid the ones that can mess up the diet. Food selection is even more important with the ketogenic diet because the wrong foods will bring ketosis to a halt.

This chapter is going to look at some of the foods that are allowed on the ketogenic diet, while showing some that you must avoid at all costs! Remember that for this dieting plan to be effective, you will have to be strict in the beginning. Any deviation can push your body out of ketosis.

Low-Carb Foods

These foods will stick to the strict 5 percent carbohydrate allowance that is allowed on the ketogenic diet.

Protein-based foods: You should try to stick to grass-fed, organic meat whenever possible. Most meats do not have added sugar, so they can be consumed in small quantities. Just remember that you cannot consume too much protein.

Fats and oils: Most of your fat should come from natural sources like nuts and meat. Supplement recipes with fats like coconut oil, butter, and olive oil.

Vegetables: You are allowed to eat both fresh and frozen vegetables. Just make sure that they are not heavy in carbs.

Foods to Get You Into Ketosis

Dairy: You are allowed to consume most dairy products, as long as they are the full fat versions.

Beverages: You will want to stick with mostly water, but the occasional stevia-based drink is okay.

Fats and Oils

Fats are going to comprise the majority of your calorie intake as you progress through the ketogenic diet. You will need to make choices based on your likes and dislikes. Unlike many other diets, you will not be forced to eat foods that you dislike. The keto diet can be customized in many different ways. For example, you can add sauces, dressing, and even butter to your meal to make it tastier.

Just keep in mind that the wrong types of fats can be extremely unhealthy. As you choose foods for your recipes, make sure that you keep an eye on the labels so you know what types of fat you are adding to your table.

> **Saturated fat:** It's okay to eat these.

> **Monounsaturated fat:** It's okay to eat these.

> **Polyunsaturated fat:** There are actually two different types of polyunsaturated fat. The kind found in fish and animal protein are healthy, but the kind found in margarine spreads are unhealthy.

> **Trans fat:** Avoid this type of fat.

Here are some great sources of healthy fats. Remember, always choose organic and grass-fed when possible:

> Fatty fish

- Lard

- Animal fat

- Mayonnaise

- Coconut butter

- Tallow

- Avocados

- Egg yolks

- Macadamia/brazil nuts

- Butter/ghee

- Cocoa butter

- Avocado oil

- Macadamia oil

- MCT oil

- Olive oil

- Coconut oil

Protein-Based Foods

Now we're going to take a closer look at protein-based foods and their impact on the ketogenic diet. It's worth noting that the higher the protein, the less you will consume. Furthermore, it's also a good idea to avoid steroids and hormone intake by choosing organic, grass-fed meats when possible.

Foods to Get You Into Ketosis

For example, dark meat poultry is much fattier than white meat, so you should choose it when possible. Fatty fish is also a great choice for the keto diet.

With red meat, you only have to worry about avoiding cured meats and sausages since they have added sugars. If you like hamburgers, then choose the fattier ground beef.

The main concern here is to make sure that you don't overdo it with protein. Too much will mess up your body's production of ketones. Furthermore, increased protein consumption can lead to the production of glucose in the body. When your goal is to reach ketosis, the production of glucose is something you absolutely do not want.

You should balance out your protein with fatty side dishes to make up the difference. For instance, if you want some beef jerky, then you should pair it with fatty cheese.

Here are some examples of protein-based foods that you can pair with the keto diet:

> **Fish:** Anything caught in the wild is preferable. The farrier, the better.

> **Shellfish:** Clams, oysters, and lobster are great addition.

> **Whole eggs:** Free-range is the best choice. Remember that you should include the yoke.

> **Beef:** Grass-fed beef when possible. Choose fattier cuts.

> **Pork:** Watch out for pork with added sugar. Also, try sticking to fattier cuts.

- ➤ **Poultry:** Again, dark meats are preferable since they contain more fat.

- ➤ **Other meats:** Veal and lamb are two great choices. Just make sure to stick with the fattier cuts.

- ➤ **Bacon/Ssausage:** Anything that is cured or contains sugars should be avoided.

Vegetables and Fruits

Here is a list of foods that can be consumed on the ketogenic diet. You will want to stay away from selections that have a high amount of carbs. Veggies are the foundation of the keto diet. You'll be eating a lot of them, but the problem is that there are a few healthy foods that are high in sugars. While they are certainly healthy, they are not going to work with the ketogenic diet, so you need to avoid them.

Your best choices are vegetables that are high in nutrients and low in carbohydrates. As you might have guessed, these are the dark, leafy vegetables. Anything that looks like spinach or kale will fall under this category.

Basically, any vegetable that is grown above ground is going to be low in carbs, but leafy, green veggies are the best. You should also try to find organic whenever possible because they contain fewer pesticides. However, organic is not an absolute necessity on the keto diet. It's just an added bonus.

There is no difference in the nutritional values of organic and non-organic vegetables. All you are doing is avoiding added chemicals like pesticides. With that said, both frozen and fresh veggies are okay.

Foods to Get You Into Ketosis

It's also worth noting that vegetables that grow below ground can still be consumed in moderation, as long as the overall macro of the recipe stays on track. Usually, vegetables that grow underground are used to add flavor to meals. Again, the key is to carefully monitor every food that you are putting into your body. Stay away from carbs whenever possible.

With vegetables, you should always keep a close eye on what you're putting into your recipes. Many people make the mistake of eating all vegetables without looking because they are "healthy," but you have to make sure your macros stays within tolerance. Pay close attention to these vegetables and fruits.

> **Higher carb veggies:** Onions, garlic, and even squash are all vegetables that you must pay very close attention to due to their high carb content.

> **Nightshades:** Eggplant, peppers, and tomatoes are all high carb veggies and should be used sparingly.

> **Berries:** While berries are very healthy foods, they also contain sugars. So you must consume them in moderation.

> **Citrus:** Lemon, lime, and orange juice – even if splashed in water – can add up quickly.

Always avoid starchy vegetables and fruits like bananas and potatoes.

Dairy Products

Now let's move onto dairy products. Most of these products are completely okay to consume on the ketogenic diet, as long as you choose the full fat options. Just keep an eye on the labels and avoid dairy that's high in carbs.

Dairy is usually added to recipes in the ketogenic diet. Just try to keep your dairy consumption in moderation. Most meals are going to come mostly from protein, vegetables, and fats.

If they are available, you should try sticking with organic and raw dairy products. Dairy that's highly processed will have two to five times the number of carbohydrates as their raw counterparts. Again, you should avoid low-fat or fat-free options since they use carbs to add in flavor.

Those with lactose sensitivities should consume hard, long-aged products since they contain a lot less lactose. Here are a few examples of dairy products that you can eat on the ketogenic diet.

➢ Greek yogurt

➢ Heavy whipping cream

➢ Cottage cheese, cream cheese, sour cream, and other spreadable dairies.

➢ Soft cheeses like mozzarella, brie, and Monterey Jack are all keto friendly.

➢ Hard cheeses like aged cheddar, Parmesan, and Swiss are all great choices for a keto-friendly lifestyle.

➢ Full fat mayonnaise. Just make sure you pay attention to the label to ensure there are no added sugars.

Dairy is an amazing way of adding extra fat into meals, but it also has protein, which you have to keep in mind. This is an important consideration when pairing dairy with protein-rich recipes.

Foods to Get You Into Ketosis

Nuts and Seeds

Now it's time we move onto another of the foundational foods of the ketogenic diet. Nuts and seeds are a great source of fat and are best when roasted because it removes any anti-nutrients. Also, you will need to avoid peanuts since they are a legume and are not permitted on the ketogenic diet food list.

Typically, nuts are a great way to flavor meals while also adding in some much needed fat. Their main role in the keto diet is in making fat bombs, a food that we'll discuss in greater detail later in this book.

Always remember that nuts have a carb count that can add up quite quickly. Furthermore, they contain protein which, again, adds up quickly. Read labels and pay close attention to the way they affect your macros.

Nuts and seeds are high in omega 6 fatty acids, which means they should be eaten in moderation. Fattier, low carb nuts are your best choice for the keto diet.

Here are some facts that you need to keep in mind about the different types of nuts:

> **Fatty, low carbohydrate nuts:** Macadamia nuts, Brazil nuts, and pecans are all great examples of nuts that can be consumed with meals on the keto diet.

> **Fatty, moderate carbohydrate nuts:** Walnuts and almonds are two examples of this category. They can be used in moderation for added flavor or for texture.

> **High carbohydrate nuts:** Pistachios and cashews contain a high level of carbohydrates and should rarely be eaten.

Making Flours Using Nuts and Seeds

This is one of the best dieting tricks because it allows you to substitute nuts and seeds for flour. You can commonly find nut and seed flours in baking recipes. Just remember that they should be eaten in moderation.

You will normally use a mixture of multiple flours to get a desirable texture. Sometimes this requires a bit of experimentation. For example, lemon poppy seed muffins have a great texture when they are combined with fats from heavy creamer and butter.

You can also use these flours for frying foods. Or you can make a pizza. There is a lot of opportunity here to do amazing things.

Beverages

It's time to move onto beverages, one of the most difficult changes to make with any dieting plan. Did you know that most people spend their days dehydrated? When we wake up, we are normally behind on water intake and never quite make up for it throughout the day. The problem is that we simply don't drink enough water. I know, water is boring in today's culture with so many other beverages so readily available. But the truth is that no dieting plan is going to work if you do not drink the right amount of water.

When you add on the fact that the ketogenic process has a natural diuretic effect, those who are starting out are going to be even more dehydrated. If you are prone to bladder pain or urinary tract infections, then you will need to take even further steps to prepare.

The general rule of thumb is to divide your weight (in pounds) by 2. That is how many ounces of water that you should drink every day. Then add even more water to that. Most keto experts recommend up to a gallon of water per day!

Foods to Get You Into Ketosis

Keto-proof coffee is a popular choice for those on this diet because it can help ramp up those energy levels. That's a good strategy, but it's also essential that you limit your consumption of flavored beverages. Furthermore, caffeine can actually cause weight loss to stall, so you should never consume more than two cups of caffeinated beverages per day.

Important Hydration Note

A lot of individuals experience a symptom known as "keto flu" when transitioning over to the ketogenic diet. This is due to dehydration and lack of electrolytes. Therefore, you need to make sure that you drink plenty of water and replenish your electrolytes. You can replenish electrolytes by drinking bone broth or sports drinks that are sweetened with sucralose or stevia.

Here are some of the common beverages that are consumed on the keto diet:

➤ **Water:** This is going to be your main source of hydration. If you must have flavor, then you can drink sparkling water.

➤ **Broth:** It's loaded with vitamins and minerals. Plus it replenishes your electrolytes. Just be sure to read the label to make sure there is no added sugar.

➤ **Coffee:** Coffee actually possesses a few weight loss benefits, as long as it's consumed in moderation. It also improves mental focus.

➤ **Tea:** Tea has the same effect as coffee, as long as you stick with black or green tea.

- **Coconut/almond milk:** You can choose to replace your normal dairy beverage with an unsweetened version that's found in a carton.

- **Diet soda:** You should avoid diet beverages because they can lead to sugar cravings and insulin spikes.

- **Water flavoring:** Small packets that are flavored using sucralose or stevia are okay on the keto diet. You can even squeeze a little lemon, lime, or orange juice into your water.

- **Alcohol:** If you are out and want a drink, then choose hard liquor. Just remember that consuming too much alcohol will actually hinder your weight loss.

Spices and Cooking in a Keto-Friendly Way

It's time we move onto cooking in a way that fits the keto lifestyle. Even small ingredients can rack up the carbs, so you must pay close attention to what you're cooking with.

Seasonings and sauces can be quite tricky when cooking in a keto-friendly manner. People use them regularly to add flavor to their food. So the first piece of advice that I can give you–and perhaps the most important–is that you should always avoid processed foods.

There are too many low carb condiments to list here. However, the majority of them use glycemic index sweeteners. You want to avoid those!

Also keep in mind that spices have carbs in them, so you need to make sure that you add them to your overall counts.

Sea salt is always preferable to table salt, since it is usually mixed with powdered dextrose.

Foods to Get You Into Ketosis

Most premade spices will have added sugars, so you will need to pay close attention to nutritional labels. Never include added sugars to your meals unless you have no other choice.

Here are some of the common herbs and spices that are keto-friendly. Some of these spices do contain carbs so you need to add them into your macros.

- ➤ Sea salt
- ➤ Black pepper
- ➤ Cayenne pepper
- ➤ Chili powder
- ➤ Oregano
- ➤ Basil
- ➤ Cilantro
- ➤ Rosemary
- ➤ Thyme
- ➤ Cinnamon
- ➤ Cumin
- ➤ Parsley

Condiments and Sauces

The next step of our keto journey takes us down the condiments and sauce aisle. You must always pay close attention to labels because some sauces can contain surreal amounts of sugar in a single teaspoon. Make sure that it fits in with your macros before you include it in recipes.

There is a significant gray area when it comes to sauces and condiments. If you want to be strict and experience better results, then you will need to stick with the ones listed below and avoid all other premade sauces. Since many of them will have added sugars that can really mess up ketosis.

With that in mind, you can be a bit less strict and use other sauces and condiments as long as you make sure that they fit your macros.

If you do choose to make your own sauces, then you should invest in a guar or xanthan gum. It's a great addition to any low carb cooking technique because it thickens sauces that might otherwise be watery. Fortunately, there are a lot of sauces that you can choose from that are high in fat and low in carbs–the perfect fit for your keto journey.

Another thing about condiments is that they vary by brand, so be sure to read the nutritional labels before buying them. Here are some premade condiments that can be used:

> Ketchup: Choose brands that have no added sugar.

> Mustard

> Hot sauce

> Mayonnaise

> Sauerkraut: Choose brands that have no added sugar.

> Relish: Choose brands that have no added sugar.

> Horseradish

Foods to Get You Into Ketosis

> ➢ Worcestershire sauce

> ➢ Salad dressings: Make sure you stay away from the low-fat types. Opt for fattier types of dressing.

You should always be cautious when choosing to use premade condiments with your keto-friendly meals. Always double check the nutritional label.

Sweeteners

It's time to dive into one of the common topics that so many people starting out on their keto journey ask about. Are sweeteners okay? If so, then what sweeteners should be used?

First of all, I understand that water is boring in today's society, but avoiding it is also one of the habits that you'll need to break. Water is essential to all diets. With that said, you can certainly splurge every now and then by using a sweetener to spice up your water, but moderation is important.

Stay away from anything that tastes sweet because it will help keep your sugar cravings at a minimum. Sugar cravings are a common problem that those new to the keto journey must face.

Try to find liquid sweeteners since they don't have added binders like maltodextrin and dextrose. These can add up in carbs very quickly! For keto dieting, you will need to stick with sweeteners that have a lower glycemic index.

Most of you will find that stevia and erythritol are a great way to create delicious keto-friendly desserts. If you find something that better suits your tastes, then just be sure to check out the label to make sure it's an acceptable sweetener. Typically, you want to steer clear of brands that use the fillers mentioned above (maltodextrin and dextrose).

Many low-carb products use sugar alcohols. While they claim to be "sugar free," they have the same effect on our body as sugar, so you have to avoid them.

In short, sweeteners all have a glycemic index. The higher the glycemic index, the more it will spike your blood sugar levels.

Here is a list of recommended sweeteners:

> **Stevia:** This is one of the most common sugar substitutes in the world. It has a low glycemic index, yet it's incredibly sweet. You should stick to the liquid version.

> **Sucralose:** This is a very sweet sugar substitute, but there is a lot of myths surrounding it. For instance, many people confuse sucralose with Splenda. They are actually quite different. Remember to stick with the liquid version.

> **Erythritol:** This is an amazing sugar substitute that comes with zero glycemic impact! It passes all of the way through our body without digesting; therefore, we do not absorb the carbs.

> **Monk fruit:** Here, we have a sweetener that is not so commonly known. It's normally used in conjunction with other sweeteners. It can serve as a balanced sweetener.

>

Sugar Addiction

Most of the cravings we get are caused by sugar. In short, the entire sugar industry is run on addiction. It's probably the biggest addition in the world and arguably the most dangerous. Consuming sugar stimulates the reward sections of the brain.

When we consume sugar, dopamine is released in our brain–the same thing that happens to individuals who use drugs. Dopamine makes us feel amazing, so it becomes quite addicting. Furthermore, the tolerance increases over time, requiring more sugar to make us feel happy.

Once the body becomes dependent on this chemical reaction, we'll start craving sugar even when we're not hungry. When shifting from a high carb diet to the ketogenic lifestyle, you are going to experience sugar cravings. That means you will need to clear out your home of sweets before you start.

In fact, I highly recommend that you restrict sweeteners for the first month so that you can completely break your sugar addiction. Trust me, you will feel amazing once this addiction has been broken.

Finding Hidden Carbs

Starting on your keto journey can be difficult in the earliest stages. Understanding what to eat and what not to eat will take practice. That's why this chapter on food is so long. I want to assure you that if you make a few mistakes in the beginning, then you are going to be okay. It happens. Learn a lesson and move forward. I can't tell you how many people give up after making a mistake.

In some cases, it's not even your fault at all. Some companies are really good at hiding their unhealthy foods behind fancy packaging. Here are some of the items that you need to look out for. If a label claims this, then it could potentially have hidden carbs.

Low-carb products: There are a bunch of products that are labeled as "low carb." Snack bars are one example. It's best to stay away from these products. At the very least, you need to read the label because they tend to use high index glycemic sweeteners.

Spices: All spices have carbs but some have more carbs than others. For example, onion powder, garlic powder, and ginger are all high carb spices. You need to make sure you read labels and use spices that contain no added sugars.

Fruits/berries: You are not allowed to consume most fruits while on the ketogenic diet because they are loaded with sugar. You can eat berries, but only in moderation. My point is that fruits might be "healthy," but they are not compatible with the ketogenic diet.

Tomato-based products: Be absolutely sure to read labels before you use tomato sauces or diced canned tomatoes. Serving sizes are important here because companies tend to use smaller serving sizes to make their foods appear healthier. Furthermore, make sure there are no added sugars.

Condiments: Adding sauce to recipes is almost a tradition today. Just be careful since many condiments hide their carbs behind minuscule serving sizes.

Peppers: Peppers can sometimes contain a lot of sugar. For example, a tiny chili pepper contains up to 4g of carbs! Bell peppers have an even higher amount that that!

Diet soda: You are allowed to drink diet soda on the keto diet, but you must keep it to a minimum. People have actually reportedly been kicked out of ketosis after consuming a large amount of diet soda. In fact, if you can cut it completely out, then I highly recommend doing so because there is a link between the consumption of diet soda and sugar cravings.

Foods to Get You Into Ketosis

Chocolate: Chocolate is allowed on the ketogenic diet but you have to be very careful with it. Also, stick with dark chocolate since it has fewer carbs.

Medicine: This is one hidden carb that most people don't even consider. Over-the-counter medicines can be loaded with sugar! Find sugar-free alternatives that are designed for diabetics.

The truth is that companies have gotten really good at hiding their carbs in packaging while still sticking to the written law, so you need to learn to properly read food labels. It's the only way you can be absolutely sure of the nutrients that you're putting into your body.

Foods That You Should Avoid

By this point, you have a great place to start when choosing the foods to eat during your keto journey. You'll find that practice does make you embed this list into your mind. After a bit of time, it will become second nature to you.

With that in mind, I feel that the best way to end this chapter is to list some of the foods that you should avoid at all costs. Seriously, these foods will throw your body out of ketosis almost instantly.

Sugar: Sugar is the greatest enemy to living a healthier lifestyle. This is true with any dieting plan. Soda, juice, sports drinks, candy, and ice cream are all loaded with artificial sugar and should be avoided at all costs. Processed foods are also loaded with sugar.

Grains: Wheat products like bread, pasta, cereal, and even beer should be avoided. This includes whole grains.

Starch: Vegetables like potatoes and yams contain a high amount of starch, which will throw your body out of ketosis. Some root vegetables are okay, but you will need to check out their nutritional information.

Trans fat: Avoid margarine and other spreadable butters as they contain this unhealthy type of fat. Even though we are aiming for more fat in our foods, we still need to stick to the healthier types of fat. Otherwise, we will run into other health problems in the long-term.

Low-fat foods: These are almost always higher in carbs because brands add sugar to make up for the loss in taste. Make sure you pay close attention to labels.

As a general rule of thumb, real foods are usually healthier for you. Some processed foods are acceptable, but most of them are unhealthy. That's why reading labels is so important.

Chapter 3
Fat Bombs for a Quick Energy Boost

Fat bombs are one of the staples of the ketogenic diet. They are designed to give you a quick boost of fat boosting energy to get you through those sluggish times. They are also an amazing treat!

This chapter is going to cover these amazing fat burning recipes by explaining how they work, how to make them, and even share a few recipes with you. Once you learn the secret to creating these powerful snacks, you'll be able to satisfy those afternoon cravings with relative ease.

Ketogenic fat bombs are treats that are high in fat, low in carbs, and usually very small. You can enjoy them as a quick breakfast or as an afternoon snack. They even serve as a great pre-workout booster to add extra fuel to your routine!

Let's start by looking at some facts about these fat bombs and what makes them tick.

They Are Usually Very Small

When I say small, I mean that you can usually eat them in just a couple of bites. They are high in fat, so it doesn't take much to give you that extra boost of energy. One of the best ways to prepare fat bombs is to use a muffin pan with a liner, and form them into small balls. That way, you don't even have to even get your hands dirty! Fat bombs are extremely easy to eat without making a mess, so they are a great way to make sure your metabolism is soaring even on the busiest of days.

They Can Be Sweet or Savory

Most of the fat bomb recipes that you'll create are going to be sweetened by stevia (or another healthy substitute). That's because stevia is one of the most keto-friendly substitutes on the market. However, if you do not like stevia, then you can use your own choice of low-carb sweetener. Just be sure that it does not use sugar alcohol. Finally, there are also savory fat bombs that are made of avocado or bacon.

They Should Be Loaded with Healthy Fat

Fat bombs are loaded with fat so you need to make sure that it's the healthy kind of fat. Eating healthy fat is a cornerstone of the ketogenic diet. You should use oils like coconut oil or coconut butter as an ingredient. Furthermore, coconut oil solidifies when refrigerated so it's the least messy of all oils.

Fat Bombs Are Refrigerated

Fat bombs will liquefy at room temperature since they contain so much fat, so you will need to store them in the refrigerator. They can last up to two weeks in the refrigerator, as long as they are in an airtight container. You can even go as far as to freeze them! Just be sure to thaw them out before taking a bite.

They Usually Contain Nuts and Seeds

It is recommended that you limit your nut and seed consumption while on the ketogenic diet since they can become oxidized when being cooked. Plus they are usually high in carbs. However, in limited quantity, nuts and seeds can provide a significant boost to your metabolic rate. This makes them a great choice for fat bombs!

Fat Bombs for a Quick Energy Boost

Three Easy Steps to Make Your Own Fat Bombs

Fat bombs are actually incredibly easy to make. This guide is going to show you how to make them in three easy steps, but before we get into the details, let's take a closer look at the three basic ingredients.

Healthy Fats

- Coconut oil

- Coconut butter

- Cacao butter

- Almond butter

- Ghee

- Butter (real butter, not margarine)

- Bacon fat

- Avocado oil

Flavoring

- Sugar-free vanilla extract

- Dark chocolate (100%)

- Cacao powder

- Salt

- Peppermint extract

- Spices

Texture

> Pecans

> Walnuts

> Almonds

> Cacao nuts

> Chia seeds

> Bacon bits (real, but artificial as they contain sugar)

> Shredded coconut

Those were just a few examples of possible ingredients. Here are the three steps to making keto fat bombs.

Step 1

Mix all ingredients together in a bowl or a blender. If the fat you choose to use is solid, then you will need to put it into the microwave to slightly melt it.

Step 2

Form the mixture into small balls. You can either use your hands, or pour the mixture onto a lined baking pan.

Step 3

Refrigerate the mixture for several hours until it's solid. If you used a baking pan, then you will need to cut the mixture into small portions.

Fat Bombs for a Quick Energy Boost

As you can see, this process is very straight-forward. Coming up with your own recipes is where things get a bit more complicated. That's why I'm going to share a few with you now.

Four Amazing Fat Bomb Recipes!

Coconut Berry Delights

Ingredients

> ➢ 1 Cup coconut oil

> ➢ ½ Cup mixed berries, frozen or fresh

> ➢ 1 Tsp. vanilla extract

> ➢ 14 drops of Sweetleaf liquid stevia (you may substitute this with honey)

Instructions

1. Melt coconut oil in the microwave on the stove. While melting, place the berries in a food processor until they have been chopped into very small pieces.

2. Add in the vanilla extract and Stevia to the food processor with the berry mixture.

3. Mix the coconut oil into the food processor. Then, process the ingredients until everything has been smoothly blended together.

4. This mix will now be thickly blended, so you can scoop up the mixture with a spoon and drop them on a parchment-lined surface. You can also use molds if you want these snacks to look prettier.

5. Place the fat bombs into the refrigerator. Once they have become solid, move them to an air-tight container.

Macro (per bomb)

Calories: 121

Fat Bombs for a Quick Energy Boost

Fat: 14g.

Net Carbs: 1g.

Protein: 0g.

Chocolate Peanut Butter Fat Bombs

Ingredients

Layer 1: Chocolate

> ➤ 2 Tbsp. coconut oil
>
> ➤ 4 Tbsp. peanut butter
>
> ➤ 4 Tbsp. cocoa powder, unsweetened
>
> ➤ ¼ Tsp. vanilla extract
>
> ➤ ¼ Tsp. stevia, liquid

Layer 2: Peanut Butter

> ➤ 2 Tbsp. coconut oil
>
> ➤ 4 Tbsp. almond butter or peanut butter
>
> ➤ ¼ Tsp. vanilla extract
>
> ➤ ¼ Tsp. stevia, liquid

Instructions

Layer 1: Chocolate

1. Mix together all ingredients until they are smooth.

2. Pour this mixture into muffin cups. Place in freezer for 10 minutes.

Layer 2: Peanut Butter

1. Mix all ingredients together

2. Pour mixture on top of chocolate layer.

3. Place in the refrigerator until firm. Then swap over to an air tight container.

Macro (per bomb)

Calories: 128

Fat: 12g.

Net Carbs: 2g.

Protein: 3g.

Amazing Almond Bombs

Ingredients

- ➤ 4 Tbsp. coconut butter

- ➤ 4 Tbsp. almond butter

- ➤ 1 Oz. cocoa powder

- ➤ 2 Tbsp. sugar free syrup

- ➤ 16 G. dark chocolate

Instructions

Fat Bombs for a Quick Energy Boost

1. Mix all ingredients together, except for the coconut butter.

2. Microwave the mixture for 15 seconds, stirring. Repeat this until all of the ingredients have been fully incorporated together.

3. Mix in coconut butter until everything is well-blended.

4. Use a spoon to divide out the mixture into a dozen or so portions. Use a lined tray.

5. Place bombs in the refrigerator until they are solid, then move them to an airtight container.

Macro (per bomb)

Calories: 100

Fat: 12g.

Net Carbs: 2g.

Protein: 2g.

Vanilla Chocolate Cheesecake Bombs

Ingredients

Bottom Layer

> ➢ 150 G. cream cheese

> ➢ 50 g. melted butter

> ➢ 1 Tbsp. Natvia

> ➢ 1 Tsp. vanilla extract

> ➢ ¼ Cup coconut oil

Top Layer

> ➢ ½ Cup coconut oil

> ➢ 1 Tsp. cocoa powder

> ➢ 2 Tsp. Natvia

Instructions

Bottom Layer

1. Mix together butter and cream cheese until they have been thoroughly combined.

2. Add in vanilla, coconut oil, and Natvia. Mix.

3. Place evenly into a cupcake tray, layering it into approximately a dozen sections.

4. Smooth the top and place in the freezer until solid.

Top Layer

1. Mix together the coconut oil, cocoa powder, and Natvia.

2. Pour this mixture on top of the hardened layers. Place in the freezer for 4 hours.

Macro (per bomb)

Calories: 312

Fat: 32g.

Net Carbs: 1g.

Fat Bombs for a Quick Energy Boost

Protein: 3g.

Chapter 4
Macros and the Ketogenic Diet

I have used the word "macros" a lot through this book, so now it's time to go into a little more detail about how it works. This might seem mind-boggling to some of you who are just starting your keto journey, but it's really not that bad. So my goal is to make this as simple as possible.

The term "macros" stands for "macronutrients." These are the components of food that provide energy to our body. Carbs, protein, and fat are where calories are derived.

There, doesn't that make you feel a little more comfortable? The truth is that with any diet, you have to understand the importance of macros because they must be included in a balanced way. With the ketogenic diet, you absolutely must pay close attention to your macros because the entire concept is dependent on staying in ketosis. While minor slip ups will not derail you, consistently enforcing the wrong macros will hinder your fat burning efforts.

Now let's take a closer look at the three components of macros.

Carbohydrates

Carbohydrates are not essential to survival. They are, in fact, the only macronutrient to hold that distinction. Carbs are comprised of fatty acids and amino acids. Made up of sugars and starches, carbs will keep the body from reaching a state of ketosis so the whole goal of this dieting plan is to limit them.

Also note that fiber is also considered a carb, but it does not count against your ketosis goal. We cannot digest fiber so it has very little impact on our blood sugar level.

Macros and the Ketogenic Diet

So when looking at a food label, you can subtract the "fiber" from the "total carbs" to determine your macro carb content. This number is known as the net carb count.

When you are looking at a nutrition label, look at the line that says "total carbs," then to the line that says "fiber." Subtract the fiber from the total carbs to calculate your net carb count.

Net carbs are nothing but wasteful carbs–sugar and starch–so it's the only number that matters for our macros. The takeaway here is that "total carbs" are not what you need to track. "Net carbs" are the important ones.

In order to successfully navigate the path to ketosis, you have to identify the foods that are low in carbohydrates so that you know what to avoid. Always check nutritional labels. Never trust the words "low carbs" or "healthy" on the front.

Protein

The body uses protein for growth, muscle regeneration, tissue repair, immune operation, and preserving muscle mass. In short, it plays a pivotal role in your biological processes. In fact, proteins are the building blocks of the body.

The body will break down protein into amino acids, many of which cannot be created any other way. These are essential to the overall function of the body. Malnutrition is one of the results of protein deficiency.

When on the ketogenic diet, you will need to consume enough protein to stay healthy while making sure to keep the count low enough so that it doesn't break ketosis.

You do not want to lose your lean muscle mass! Many people head into a diet with the goal of losing weight, but really you want to lose fat. Muscle mass has a lot of healthy benefits, including the fact that it boosts your metabolism. So it's important that you shift your metabolism.

Your macros should include a healthy level of protein, but not too much.

Fats

Our body needs a certain amount of fat for energy, growth and development. It's essential to absorbing vitamins and even helps to maintain cell membranes. There's a reason why our body finds fats so delicious.

Fat is extremely satisfying to the body, so being able to consume it on a diet is a godsend! That's why the ketogenic diet has been so successful. Imagine being able to fill your body with fat while still losing weight. That is how the keto diet works.

If you are keeping your carbs to a minimum and eating just enough protein to preserve your lean muscle, then consuming fat actually transforms your body into a fat burning machine.

That's not saying that you don't have to watch your calorie count. You will need to consume fewer calories than your body burns throughout the day. This varies depending on a number of factors.

Calculating Macros

Calculating macros is all based on the information we just reviewed. I recommend you use a calculator, but it's still essential that you understand how they work. Here is an example of how you would manually calculate macros.

Macros and the Ketogenic Diet

Let's say that we have a guy named Thomas. He is a 160 pound guy who is looking to lose fat. He is 5 foot 4 inches, doesn't exercise, and has an office job. He also has about 30 percent body fat right now.

You'll find that the following are true:

Thomas has a base metabolic rate of 1,467 calories.

Thomas has a daily energy expenditure of 1,614 calories.

When we plug this information into a macro calculator, we discover that his macro is as follows:

- Fat: 86 grams (774 calories)

- Carbs: 20 grams (80 calories)

- Protein: 90 grams (360 calories)

This macro is 72 percent fat, 5 percent carbs, and 23 percent protein. It also has a calorie deficit based on his daily expenditure.

Just remember that as you lose weight, your body will change, so you will need to recalculate your macros. If you fail to keep your macros up-to-date, then you might stall ketosis.

Also, keep in mind that if Thomas had different goals other than fat loss, then his macro would have been different.

As a summary, when you "track your macros," you are actually doing the following:

Define Your Health Goals: Write down your overall health goals. Are you looking to lose fat? Build muscle mass? Or do you just want to start eating a healthier diet?

Fat, Carbs, and Protein: Determining the amount of each nutrient to include in your diet is an essential step in achieving your health goals.

Calculate Meals: You need to calculate each recipe, and write down their macros. That way, you can keep track of the foods you're consuming.

Create a Meal Plan: Based on the recipes you create, you will need to form your meal plan for each day. I recommend you do this a week at a time.

The truth is that tracking your macros every day is going to get very stressful. It's much easier to plan your meals ahead of time. Then you can shop based on that plan. It's a stress-free way that makes it easier to stick with your dieting plan.

Macro Calculators

Keto calculators will help you determine the number of fat, carbs, and protein you will need to consume in order to meet your goals. Here are three of the best online calculators that I have found.

https://www.perfectketo.com/keto-macro-calculator/

https://www.ruled.me/keto-calculator/

https://ketodietapp.com/Blog/page/KetoDiet-Buddy

Chapter 5
Exercising While in Ketosis

Getting your body into ketosis means that you are ridding it of carbs—the source of fuel that it has been accustomed to using your whole life. That means exercise is going to be a bit tricky at first, but that doesn't mean that it's impossible.

It's important that you understand the misconceptions around the link between a low-carb diet and exercise. Let's start by looking at the traditional view of weight loss. People see losing weight as eating less and exercising more. That is just too vague to be sustainable.

In order to experience long-term results, you will need to be cautious about what you put into your body. You cannot out exercise a bad diet.

This is one of the reasons why the ketogenic diet is so successful. So first and foremost, you need to be strict about what you consume. That is far more important than exercise.

With that said, including exercise as part of your keto journey can significantly boost your overall success. It's good for your heart and helps you build lean muscles. This chapter is going to show you the types of exercises you can fit into your overall keto routine.

The Four Types of Exercise That Best Compliment the Ketogenic Diet

Your nutritional needs will vary depending on the type of exercise you are performing. Since we're using a diet-first approach, you'll need to plan the type of exercise you do around your health goals.

Aerobic Exercise

Some people call this cardio exercise. The two are the same type of exercise. Aerobic exercise is anything that lasts over three minutes. Since aerobic exercise is very low intensity, it's very friendly to the keto dieter.

Anaerobic Exercise

This type of exercise utilizes short bursts of energy. For example, high-intensity weight training is a type of anaerobic exercise. Carbohydrates are used by the body as the primary source of fuel for this type of workout, so keto dieters should stay away from it.

Flexibility Exercises

Flexibility exercises are an amazing way to stretch out your muscles and improve their range. In fact, improving your flexibility can help you prevent injuries by shortening the muscles. Yoga is the most popular example of flexibility exercise.

Stability Exercises

This includes any type of balance and core training exercises. They will help you improve your strength, control, and alignment. This is another good exercise for those on the keto diet.

The key to exercising while on the ketogenic diet is to understand that your body is relying on fat as a primary source of fuel. Workout intensity matters a lot when in ketosis:

> ➤ The body uses fat as a primary fuel source during low-intensity workouts.

> ➤ The body uses carbohydrates as a primary source of fuel during high-intensity workouts.

Exercising While in Ketosis

That tells us that we need to stay away from high-intensity workouts since they rely on carbohydrates. So we're going to target our exercise around the ketogenic diet.

How to Target Ketogenic Dieting to Our Exercise

Some of you who are reading this book might perform exercises that are more intense, like weightlifting more than three days per week. If so, then you can actually adjust your carbs to match this type of high-intensity exercise. What most people do is they eat some king of fast-acting carb 30 minutes before their high-intensity workout. Fruit is usually the carb of choice here. This makes sure that your body gets enough glycogen to fuel your muscles during your high-intensity workout. If done this way, your body will not leave ketosis since the carbs are being burned immediately.

Ketogenic Adaptation

It takes your body approximately two to three weeks to adapt to a low-carb diet, so it's important that you understand how your body reacts to the change in its primary fuel source. Even though the body prefers glycogen as its primary fuel source, the longer you remain on the ketogenic diet, the more adaptive your body will be. It will start to become more efficient during exercise.

Why Exercise is Beneficial for Ketosis

Some people say that ketosis will hinder a long-term workout plan, but that is not the truth. In fact, there are a lot of benefits to combining ketosis with regular exercise.

➢ You will burn even more fat by combining low-intensity aerobic exercise with the ketogenic diet.

➢ Ketosis helps prevent fatigue during longer periods of aerobic exercise.

> Obese individuals will experience better blood glucose maintenance during exercise.

> Over time, the body adapts to a low-carb diet during exercise.

Best Exercise for Keto Dieters

Cardio workouts are the absolute best way to approach the ketogenic diet. As you are adapting to this new lifestyle, you will want to keep your intensity at roughly 50 percent and gradually increase it. This helps your body adapt to ketosis. You will gradually increase your cardio workouts by 5 minutes each week until you have reached the 45 minute mark. Here are some of the best exercises:

> Running

> Cycling

> Interval Training

> Recreational Sports

> Swimming

Your strength might feel as if it's decreasing in the beginning due to your carb restrictions, but it will gradually build back up. There is no reason to push yourself. We're aiming for low-intensity workouts.

My point is that exercising while following the ketogenic diet requires you to be mindful of the exercises you choose.

Chapter 6
Staying Motivated

You probably know now that the ketogenic journey is one of the most effective paths to weight loss. It helps you lose weight while feeling healthy, experiencing no cravings, and eating many of the foods you enjoy. As with all other diets, there are restrictions in what you can eat. Those restrictions can be frustrating, and there are going to be times when it's extremely difficult.

So now I'm going to wrap up this book by sharing some tips to help keep your motivation at an all-time high.

Support Makes the Journey Easier

Every journey you take is much easier in groups. If you have friends who also want to get into shape and live a healthier life, then you should encourage them to join you on your journey. That way, you can experience the highs and lows together. Plus, you can have fun exercising together and experiencing new, delicious recipes.

If you don't know anyone in person who wants to share in your journey, then you can find a great deal of support online. The ketogenic diet is quite popular so there are a lot of forums dedicated to people having discussions about it. You can use these as inspiration and as you meet more people, you can create groups that share common goals.

Focus on Positives Rather Than Negatives

If you find yourself craving a Little Debbie snack cake, then focus on the positives of what you have already achieved. I am not just talking about the weight you might have lost by this point, but the overall positive impact the keto diet has had on your overall health.

Do you have more energy than you used to? Are you sleeping better? Consider how you feel now compared to how you used to feel when being bogged down with carbs.

Is it worth setting yourself back just to enjoy a temporary pleasure?

Deal with Setbacks Immediately

If you have a setback, don't panic! It's bound to happen, and the worst thing you can do is panic. The keto journey is a lifestyle change, so it's unrealistic to expect there to be no mistakes. You're sure to fall prey to temptation. Just remember that when you consume a high amount of carbs, your body will fall out of ketosis. It takes a couple of days to get yourself back on track, but you should start immediately. Brush yourself off, and get back to it!

Learn from your mistakes to ensure that it doesn't happen again.

Start Your Day on a Positive Note

There are hundreds of motivational quotes that can help you start your day off on a positive note. It's amazing at how starting your day off with optimism will improve your entire day. Try it! You will be amazed at the results.

There are also affirmations that you can repeat every morning that will help get you on the right track. Some examples include:

"I prefer foods that are healthier for my body."

"I look forward to another day of living a healthier life."

Staying Motivated

"I am going to return my body to its optimal health by giving it what it needs."

Develop a morning routine that is designed to promote positivity. Mindset goes a long way!

Continuously Educate Yourself About Health

I encourage you to read something health-related every day, whether it be a success story of someone on the ketogenic diet, or an amazing new keto study. Maybe you could even read about new recipes.

Even though you might not be an avid fan of science, it's still good to learn why the ketogenic diet works. It's also quite inspiring when you understand that society is bombarded with the false belief that fat is bad and that fat is what causes us to gain weight. That's really not the truth. What causes us to gain weight is consuming more calories than we burn. Ketosis makes sure that we are burning more calories, but we still have to stay at a calorie deficit.

As a final note, there is never a scenario where you "have no choice" but to eat an unhealthy food. I mean, assuming no one is holding a gun to your head, you always have a choice. Once you understand just how powerful the ketogenic diet is and how much more amazing it will make you feel, the excuses will stop. You will replace those excuses with action!

Everyone has their breaking point—a point when they reach rock bottom and are forced to make a change. I hope you never find yours, but even if you do, here are some final words of encouragement. As ugly as rock bottom might be, it's one of the greatest motivators to change.

Final Thoughts

The ketogenic diet exists in a world of its own. It combines the powerful effects of calorie restriction with the added benefits of putting your body into ketosis. It's one of the most successful weight loss methods in existence right now.

With that said, I feel that many people seem to believe everything that they read online, so there is a bit of discrepancy between myths and scientific facts as to what's the healthiest choice. Some myths include:

I will lose weight as long as I stay in ketosis.

Carbs are the only reason I am gaining weight.

Calories don't matter on the ketogenic diet.

These are all untrue. In order to lose weight, you must be at a calorie deficit. In other words, you will always gain weight if you consume more calories than you burn. As far as carbs being the main reason for weight gain, athletes are required to consume carbs because of their workout regimen, yet they seem to be in wonderful shape.

The reason ketosis works for the average person is because most people are not exercising four plus hours per day. The average person does not have a personal trainer calculating all of their intake and creating workout plans based around their dieting plan. Most people need to find alternate methods of boosting their metabolism—to make their body work for them.

That's why I am ending this book with a few tips that should clear up some of these misconceptions.

Final Thoughts

- Calories do matter. You need to use a macro calculator to determine how many calories you consume in a given day.

- You must be strict with the foods you consume. Even one cheat day will throw you out of ketosis.

- You have to read labels carefully.

- Keep a food journal to track your macros.

- Take charge of your food environment. Do not keep carb heavy foods in your home. Temptation can get the best of you, so it's best to remove it.

- Collaborate with other people who share similar goals.

- Stay hydrated to avoid the keto flu.

Four-Week
Ketogenic
Meal
Plan

Meal Plan Introduction

This section is going to show you a four-week meal plan that will help make your keto journey much easier to start. Here are some key tips to keep in mind.

1. Make sure that you read labels carefully. Even though the label says "zero carbs" there might be sugar alcohol or something else hidden in the ingredients that can actually cause you to fall out of ketosis.

2. You will have leftovers that are used in some meals. It gives you a break from having to cook every day.

3. You must track your calories, and always stay under your recommend daily count. Remember that you can only lose weight when you are at a calorie deficit.

4. Remember that exercise is a bonus and will help lead you towards a healthier lifestyle. But it is not a requirement.

Week 1

Monday

Breakfast: Ultimate Breakfast Roll Ups

Lunch: Ultimate Breakfast Roll Ups

Afternoon Snack: Amazing Almond Bombs

Dinner: Amazing Keto Meatballs

Tuesday

Breakfast: Amazing Almond Bombs

Lunch: Amazing Keto Meatballs

Dinner: Beef and Veggie Stir-Fry

Wednesday

Breakfast: Mini Pizza Egg Bakes

Lunch: Mini Pizza Egg Bakes

Afternoon Snack: Amazing Almond Bombs

Dinner: Beef and Veggie Stir-Fry

Thursday

Breakfast: Baked Eggs with Cheesy Hash

Lunch: Amazing Almond Bombs

Final Thoughts

Dinner: Bacon Cheeseburger Casserole

Friday

Breakfast: Baked Eggs with Cheesy Hash

Lunch: Amazing Almond Bombs

Dinner: Bacon Cheeseburger Casserole

Saturday

Breakfast: Amazing Almond Bombs

Lunch: Bacon-Wrapped Chicken Bombs

Dinner: Beef Shawarma Bowl

Sunday

Breakfast: Baked Eggs with Cheesy Hash

Lunch: Bacon-Wrapped Chicken Bombs

Afternoon Snack: Amazing Almond Bombs

Dinner: Beef Shawarma Bowl

Week 2

Monday

Breakfast: Baked Eggs with Cheesy Hash

Lunch: Delicious Keto Burgers

Afternoon Snack: Vanilla Chocolate Cheesecake Bombs

Dinner: Mashed Cauliflower and Gravy

Tuesday

Breakfast: Vanilla Chocolate Cheesecake Bombs

Lunch: Delicious Keto Burgers

Dinner: Mashed Cauliflower and Gravy

Wednesday

Breakfast: Mini Pizza Egg Bakes

Lunch: Mini Pizza Egg Bakes

Afternoon Snack: Vanilla Chocolate Cheesecake Bombs

Dinner: Crustless Quiche Lorraine

Thursday

Breakfast: Baked Eggs with Cheesy Hash

Lunch: Vanilla Chocolate Cheesecake Bombs

Dinner: Crustless Quiche Lorraine

Final Thoughts

Friday

Breakfast: Baked Eggs with Cheesy Hash

Lunch: Vanilla Chocolate Cheesecake Bombs

Dinner: Spaghetti Squash Lasagna

Saturday

Breakfast: Vanilla Chocolate Cheesecake Bombs

Lunch: Spaghetti Squash Lasagna

Dinner: Creamy Beef Casserole

Sunday

Breakfast: Ultimate Breakfast Roll Ups

Lunch: Vanilla Chocolate Cheesecake Bombs

Dinner: Creamy Beef Casserole

Week 3

Monday

Breakfast: Ultimate Breakfast Roll Ups

Lunch: Chocolate Peanut Butter Fat Bombs

Dinner: Spinach Artichoke Chicken

Tuesday

Breakfast: Mini Pizza Egg Bakes

Lunch: Spinach Artichoke Chicken

Afternoon Snack: Chocolate Peanut Butter Fat Bombs

Dinner: Creamy Beef Casserole

Wednesday

Breakfast: Mini Pizza Egg Bakes

Lunch: Chocolate Peanut Butter Fat Bombs

Dinner: Creamy Beef Casserole

Thursday

Breakfast: Baked Eggs with Cheesy Hash

Lunch: Chocolate Peanut Butter Fat Bombs

Dinner: Mashed Cauliflower and Gravy

Final Thoughts

Friday

Breakfast: Baked Eggs with Cheesy Hash

Lunch: Chocolate Peanut Butter Fat Bombs

Dinner: Mashed Cauliflower and Gravy

Saturday

Breakfast: Chocolate Peanut Butter Fat Bombs

Lunch: Beef and Veggie Stir-Fry

Dinner: Delicious Keto Burgers

Sunday

Breakfast: Chocolate Peanut Butter Fat Bombs

Lunch: Delicious Keto Burgers

Dinner: Beef and Veggie Stir-Fry

Week 4

Monday

Breakfast: Baked Eggs with Cheesy Hash

Lunch: Coconut Berry Delights

Dinner: Amazing Keto Meatballs

Tuesday

Breakfast: Baked Eggs with Cheesy Hash

Lunch: Amazing Keto Meatballs

Afternoon Snack: Coconut Berry Delights

Dinner: Spaghetti Squash Lasagna

Wednesday

Breakfast: Ultimate Breakfast Roll Ups

Lunch: Coconut Berry Delights

Dinner: Spaghetti Squash Lasagna

Thursday

Breakfast: Ultimate Breakfast Roll Ups

Lunch: Spaghetti Squash Lasagna

Afternoon Snack: Coconut Berry Delights

Dinner: Delicious Keto Burgers

Final Thoughts

Friday

Breakfast: Mini Pizza Egg Bakes

Lunch: Coconut Berry Delights

Dinner: Delicious Keto Burgers

Saturday

Breakfast: Mini Pizza Egg Bakes

Lunch: Beef and Veggie Stir-Fry

Afternoon Snack: Coconut Berry Delights

Dinner: Spinach Artichoke Chicken

Sunday

Breakfast: Coconut Berry Delights

Lunch: Spinach Artichoke Chicken

Dinner: Spinach Artichoke Chicken

Recipes

Amazing Keto Meatballs

Servings: 6

Ingredients

- ✓ 1 ½ Lb. ground beef

- ✓ 1 Whole egg

- ✓ 2 Tbsp. Parmesan cheese, grated

- ✓ 1 Tbsp. flaxseed meal

- ✓ 1 Tsp. oregano, dried

- ✓ Dash of salt

- ✓ Dash of pepper

- ✓ 1 Tbsp. olive oil

- ✓ 14 Oz. can of tomato sauce (read label to make sure it has no added sugar)

Instructions

1. Mix together beef, cheese, egg, flaxseed, oregano, salt, and pepper until they have been well combined. Roll this mixture into small meatballs.

2. Add olive oil to a large skillet, and heat on medium high. Add in meatballs.

3. Cook for about 5 minutes on each side.

4. Pour tomato sauce over meatballs. Simmer for about 25 minutes.

Macros (per serving)

Calories: 444

Fat: 38g.

Net Carbs: 2g.

Protein: 36g.

Avocado Deviled Eggs

Servings: 6

Ingredients

- ✓ 6 Eggs

- ✓ 1 Avocado

- ✓ ¼ Tsp. salt

- ✓ ¼ Tsp. pepper

- ✓ ¼ Tsp. garlic

- ✓ ¼ Tsp. chili powder

- ✓ ¼ Tsp. cumin

- ✓ ¼ Tsp. paprika (optional)

- ✓ 2 Tbsp. cilantro

Instructions

1. Boil eggs in a medium pot. This will take approximately 10-15 minutes.

2. Place eggs in a bowl of ice water for 5 minutes until they are chilled.

3. Peel shells from eggs, and then cut each egg in half lengthwise. Remove the yolk.

4. Mix together the egg yolks, avocado, and all spices in a bowl.

5. Add this mixture to the egg halves, and place them onto a deviled egg tray.

6. Drizzle each deviled egg with lime juice, and sprinkle on cilantro.

Macros (per serving)

Calories: 312

Fat: 26g.

Net Carbs: 2g.

Protein: 9g.

Bacon Cheeseburger Casserole

Servings: 10

Ingredients

Beef Layer

- ✓ 1 Sliced onion

- ✓ 1 Garlic clove, crushed

- ✓ 1 ½ Lbs. ground beef

- ✓ 60 g. Full fat cream cheese

- ✓ 3 Slices bacon, diced

- ✓ Dash of sea salt

- ✓ Dash of ground black pepper

Cheese Sauce

- ✓ 3 Medium eggs

- ✓ 125 Ml. heavy cream

- ✓ 100 G. shredded cheese

- ✓ 2 Tbsp. mustard

- ✓ 2 Sliced pickles

- ✓ Dash of sea salt

✓ Dash of ground black pepper

✓ 50 G. shredded cheese (used to sprinkle over finished dish)

Instructions

Beef Layer

1. Cook bacon in a skillet until thoroughly cooked. Place to the side.

2. Using the same skillet, cook onion, garlic, and beef until it has been thoroughly cooked. Add sea salt and pepper, and then stir in the cream cheese.

3. Pour the beef mixture into a baking dish. Sprinkle it with bacon pieces.

Cheese Sauce

1. Combine eggs, cream, cheese, sea salt, pepper, and mustard in a bowl. Mix thoroughly.

2. Pour this cheese sauce over the beef and bacon mixture.

3. Add pickles over the top, and coat with the remainder of the cheese.

4. Bake at 350 degrees for 15 minutes until the cheese becomes golden. Serve this with salad.

Macros (per serving)

Calories: 613

Fat: 51g.

Recipes

Net Carbs: 3g.

Protein: 33g.

Bacon-Wrapped Chicken Bombs

Servings: 10

Ingredients

- ✓ 2 Lbs. of skinless, boneless chicken breasts
- ✓ 10 Oz. frozen spinach
- ✓ 4 Oz. softened cream cheese
- ✓ ½ Cup full-fat ricotta
- ✓ Dash of sea salt
- ✓ Dash of ground, black pepper
- ✓ 12 Slices of bacon

Instructions

1. Preheat oven to 375 Degrees.

2. Thaw spinach, and wring it to remove as much water as possible.

3. Mix together the cream cheese and ricotta. Season it with sea salt and pepper.

4. Slice the chicken in half. You will want to have thick enough slices to create pouches.

5. Cut pockets into the sliced chicken. Then stuff these pockets with cheese mixture.

6. Wrap 2 slices of bacon around each piece of chicken. Try your best to cover any holes that are remaining after cutting out the pockets.

7. Sear the chicken in a skillet just a bit. You do not have to fully cook it now, since the oven will be performing that job.

8. Place the chicken in a baking pan, and cook in the oven for 35-45 minutes. The chicken should reach 165 degrees in the center.

Macros (per serving)

Calories: 384

Fat: 20g.

Net Carbs: 2g.

Protein: 14g.

Baked Eggs with Cheesy Hash

Servings: 3

Ingredients

- ✓ 5 Oz. diced zucchini
- ✓ 6 Oz. chopped cauliflower
- ✓ ½ Red bell pepper, medium and diced
- ✓ 1 Tbsp. melted coconut oil
- ✓ 1 Tsp. smoked paprika
- ✓ 1 Tsp. onion powder
- ✓ 1 Tsp. garlic powder
- ✓ ¼ Cup Mexican blend shredded cheese
- ✓ ½ Avocado, medium
- ✓ 3 Large eggs
- ✓ 1 Tbsp. sliced jalapenos
- ✓ 3 Tbsp. cotija cheese
- ✓ 2 Tsp. Tajin seasoning

Instructions

1. Preheat oven to 400 degrees.

2. Line a baking sheet with foil, and spread zucchini, cauliflower, and red peppers evenly into baking pan. Then drizzle it with oil.

3. Sprinkle onion powder, garlic, and paprika, and then toss it all so that the seasonings blend into the mixture.

4. Bake for 15 minutes until it starts to brown.

5. Remove the vegetables from oven and then top with shredded Mexican cheese.

6. Place the avocados around the veggies, and crack 3 eggs so that they fill the spaces in between. Bake for approximately 10 minutes. Then add cotija cheese, jalapenos (optional), and Tajin on top of eggs.

Macros (per serving)

Calories: 248

Fat: 18g.

Net Carbs: 6g.

Protein: 12g.

Beef and Veggie Stir-Fry

Servings: 6

Ingredients

- ✓ 1 Lb. flank steak, sliced and trimmed

- ✓ 2 Tsp. lime juice

- ✓ 2 Tsp. coconut amino

- ✓ 2 Tbsp. avocado oil

- ✓ 3 Peeled carrots, sliced into quarter-inch pieces

- ✓ 1 Head of cabbage, thinly sliced

- ✓ 3 Fresh minced scallions

- ✓ 1 Tbsp. grated ginger

- ✓ 4 Minced garlic cloves

Sauce

- ✓ 6 Tbsp. coconut amino

- ✓ 2 Tbsp. lime juice

- ✓ 1 ½ Tsp. tapioca flour

Instructions

1. Combine steak, coconut aminos, and lime juice in a bowl. Toss to combine. Allow it to marinate for 10 minutes.

2. Heat 1 Tbsp. oil on medium in a skillet. Place half of the meat into the skille,t and cook for 1 minute on each side.

3. Place the seared steak into a bowl, and then repeat the searing process with the rest of the steak. Make sure you drain extra liquid from the skillet as required.

4. Once the meat is finished, heat the remainder of the oil in the skillet. Add carrots, and sauté for approximately 5 minutes, or until they are soft.

5. Add cabbage into the skillet, and toss it along with the carrots. Move this cabbage/carrot mixture to the side of the skillet, and sprinkle with scallions, garlic, and ginger. Stir entire contents in the center of skillet for approximately 30 seconds.

6. Toss the meat into the skillet, along with the coconut aminos, lime juice, and tapioca flour. Mix over heat until the sauce thickens, which should take no more than 2 minutes. Remove skillet from heat.

7. Divide the finished mixture in bowls that are filled with napa cabbage and garnish them with scallions.

Macros (per serving)

Calories: 376

Fat: 31g.

Net Carbs: 4g.

Protein: 21g.

Beef Satay

Servings: 6

Ingredients

Beef Satay and Marinade

- ✓ 1 Lb. flank steak
- ✓ 2 Tbsp. Red Boat fish sauce
- ✓ 2 Tbsp. soy sauce or coconut aminios
- ✓ 2 Tbsp. Swerve confection
- ✓ ½ Tsp. coriander, ground

Peanut Sauce

- ✓ ¼ Cup smooth almond butter
- ✓ 1/3 Cup coconut milk
- ✓ 1 Tsp. chile garlic sauce
- ✓ 1 Tbsp. Swerve confection
- ✓ ½ Tsp. Thai red curry paste

Other Ingredients

- ✓ 1 Tbsp. olive oil
- ✓ Bamboo skewers socked in water for at least 2 hours

Recipes

Instructions

Beef Satay

1. Cut the steak into 1 ½ inch strips. Make sure that the grain goes horizontally across the strip.

2. Place skewers into the meat so that you leave a handle long enough to hold while you're eating it.

3. Mix the fish sauce, soy sauce, and sweetener in a baking pan. Coat the surface of the steaks with this mixture.

4. Sprinkle the meat with the coriander, and then firmly rub it into the meat. Let it sit for about 20 minutes. Preheat grill while meat is marinating.

Thai Peanut Sauce

1. Warm the almond butter in the microwave for a few seconds. Then mix in the garlic sauce, sweetener, and Thai red curry paste until it's well-blended.

2. Slowly whisk in the coconut milk.

Grilling the Meat

1. Brush 1 Tbsp. of olive oil onto the meat.

2. Fold a piece of tin foil to place under handles while cooking.

3. Place meat onto the grill and cook it until done. Make sure you line the foil up under the handles.

Macros (per serving)

Calories: 373

Fat: 27g.

Net Carbs:3g.

Protein: 23g.

Recipes

Beef Shawarma Bowl

Servings: 10

Ingredients

- ✓ 1 ½ Lbs. ground beef
- ✓ 1 Tbsp. garlic powder
- ✓ 1 Tbsp. onion powder
- ✓ ½ Tbsp. cumin
- ✓ ½ Tbsp. five spice powder
- ✓ ½ Tbsp. cayenne pepper
- ✓ 1 Tsp. sea salt
- ✓ ½ Tsp. black pepper
- ✓ 2 Tbsp. Greek yogurt
- ✓ 2Tbsp. lemon juice, freshly squeezed
- ✓ 2 Tbsp. butter
- ✓ 16 Oz. cauliflower rice
- ✓ 2 Tbsp. soy sauce, light

Garlic Sauce

- ✓ 2 Tbsp. garlic powder

- ✓ ½ Tsp. onion powder

- ✓ 4 Tbsp. Greek yogurt

- ✓ ½ Tsp. sea salt

- ✓ ½ Tsp. black pepper

- ✓ 2 Tbsp. water

Red Pepper Sauce

- ✓ 1 Tsp. red pepper flakes, crushed

- ✓ 1 Tbsp. sriracha

- ✓ 1 Tbsp. chili oil

- ✓ 2 Tbsp. Greek yogurt

- ✓ ½ Tsp. sea salt

- ✓ ½ Tsp. black pepper

Instructions

Garlic Sauce

1. Mix together all ingredients into a bowl and whisk until they are well blended. You can add water for consistency. Transfer this mixture into a jar or squeeze bottle. This sauce can be stored for up to two weeks in the refrigerator.

Red Pepper Sauce

2. Mix all ingredients together in a bowl. You may add water for consistency. Transfer to a jar or squeeze bottle. This sauce can be stored for up to two weeks in the refrigerator.

Meal

3. Mix together ground beef and spices. In a separate bowl, mix together yogurt and lemon juice. Combine both mixtures together until combined and sticky.

4. Add 2 Tbsp. butter to a pan and preheat on medium. Add in the marinated beef. Cook thoroughly. Once cooked, move it to a bowl, and use foil to keep it warm.

5. Use the same pan that was used to cook the beef to prepare the cauliflower rice. Mix in the soy sauce and cook until nearly dry.

6. Layer cauliflower rice, beef, toppings, and sauces.

Macros (per serving)

Calories: 632

Fat: 46g.

Net Carbs: 15g.

Protein: 34g.

Broccoli and Chicken Casserole

Servings: 8

Ingredients

- ✓ 2 Heads of broccoli cut into florets (you can use frozen if you wish)

- ✓ 1 Large rotisserie chicken, separated from bone

- ✓ 1 Cup mayonnaise

- ✓ 2/3 Cup whipping cream, heavy

- ✓ 1 Tbsp. chicken soup base

- ✓ 1 Tbsp. dried dill weed

- ✓ 1 Tsp. ground black pepper

- ✓ 2 Cups cheddar cheese, shredded

- ✓ Cooking spray

Instructions

1. Preheat oven to 350 degrees.

2. Place broccoli florets into a baking pan. Sprinkle cheese on top, and then press down on the broccoli.

3. Mix mayonnaise, chicken soup base, dill, pepper, and heavy cream. Spread this mixture over the chicken and sprinkle shredded cheese on top of it. Place chicken into baking pan.

4. Coat a piece of aluminum foil with the cooking spray, and then cover the baking sheet, making sure the greased side is down.

5. Place baking pan in oven for approximately 45 minutes. Then remove aluminum foil and continue baking for 15 minutes. Remove from oven.

6. Let casserole stand for at least 10 minutes.

Macros (per serving)

Calories: 335

Fat: 22g.

Net Carbs: 6g.

Protein: 17g.

Bubble 'n' Squeak

Servings: 8

Ingredients

Mashed Cauliflower

- ✓ Approximately 300 g. cauliflower florets
- ✓ 2 Tbsp. heavy whipping cream
- ✓ 1 Tbsp. butter
- ✓ Dash of sea salt
- ✓ Dash of ground black pepper

Bubble n Squeak

- ✓ 3 Slices of bacon, diced
- ✓ 1 Tbsp. butter
- ✓ ¼ diced onion, medium
- ✓ 50 G. sliced leek
- ✓ 1 Stalk sliced green onion
- ✓ 50 G. chopped brussels sprouts
- ✓ ¼ Cup mozzarella, grated
- ✓ ¼ Cup Parmesan, grated

Recipes

✓ 2 Tbsp. duck fat

✓ 1 Tsp. minced garlic

Instructions

1. You can either use leftover mashed cauliflower, or place the florets into a bowl along with 1 Tbsp. butter and cream. Mix it together, and then microwave on high for approximately 4 minutes. Mix thoroughly to avoid drying out the cauliflower.

2. Place in the microwave for 4 more minutes. The cauliflower will now be soft. Season with sea salt and pepper.

3. Use a blender to finish mashing the cauliflower until it's creamy. Add mozzarella while it's still hot.

4. Put the chopped bacon into a pan, and cook on medium until it's crispy. Remove bacon and place onto a paper towel.

5. Add 1 Tbsp. butter to the bacon fat that's left in the pan. Then mix in garlic and cook it for approximately 60 seconds.

6. Add onion to the pan, and sauté for approximately 4 minutes. The onion should be translucent.

7. Add in the chopped leeks and brussels sprouts. Cook them for approximately 10 minutes or until soft.

8. Add green onions and cook for an additional minute. Remove from heat and allow the pan to cool.

9. Add bacon to the vegetable mix, and then add that new mixture to the mashed cauliflower. Season with sea salt and pepper if needed.

10. After mixing together all of the ingredients, add the duck fat. Cook in a pan on medium until it's melted. Then place the egg rings into the pan and sprinkle Parmesan into the rings.

11. Add mashed cauliflower into the rings. Sprinkle more Parmesan onto the top of it.

12. Give the mixture a chance to warm (especially if using leftovers.) Flip over and allow to cook until a crisp crust forms. Be careful that they don't get too hot, or the mixture may run. If you find they aren't crisping on the outside, turn up the heat in the pan, and press down on them for a minute or so on each side.

Macros (per serving)

Calories: 332

Fat: 28g.

Net Carbs: 8g.

Protein: 11g.

Chicken Parmesan

Servings: 4

Ingredients

- ✓ 8 Oz. chicken breast, boneless and skinless
- ✓ 1 Whole egg
- ✓ 1 Tbsp. heavy whipping cream
- ✓ 1 ½ Oz. crushed pork rinds
- ✓ 1 Oz. Parmesan cheese, grated
- ✓ ½ Tsp. salt
- ✓ ½ Tsp. black pepper, ground
- ✓ ½ Tsp. garlic powder
- ✓ ½ Tsp. red pepper flakes
- ✓ ½ Tsp. Italian seasoning
- ✓ ½ Cup tomato sauce (no added sugar)
- ✓ ¼ Cup shredded mozzarella cheese
- ✓ 1 Tbsp. ghee

Instructions

1. Place oven rack approximately 6 inches from the broiler, and preheat the oven's broiler.

2. Slice the chicken breast down the center horizontally with ½ inch of the sides. Spread them out so that you have butterfly splays. Then pound the chicken flat.

3. Mix together egg and cream.

4. Mix together pork rinds, Parmesan cheese, salt, pepper, garlic powder, red pepper, and Italian seasoning to create a breading.

5. Dip chicken into egg mixture, then thickly coat it with the breading mixture.

6. Heat a skillet over medium heat. Add in the ghee. Place chicken into the pan, and cook it until it's no longer pink in the center.

7. Place chicken onto a baking sheet. Cover with tomato sauce, and sprinkle mozzarella cheese over the top.

8. Place in oven until the cheese bubbles. This takes approximately 2 minutes.

Macros (per serving)

Calories: 350

Fat: 19g.

Net Carbs: 6g.

Protein: 18g.

Creamy Beef Casserole

Servings: 10

Ingredients

- ✓ 16 Oz. cauliflower rice

- ✓ 1.5 Lbs. ground beef

- ✓ 15 Oz. green enchilada sauce

- ✓ ½ Cup sour cream

- ✓ 1 ¼ Cups cottage cheese, small curd

- ✓ 2 Cups cheddar cheese, shredded

- ✓ ½ Cup green onion, sliced

- ✓ 1 Tsp. sea salt

- ✓ 1 Tsp. black pepper

Instructions

1. Preheat oven to 350 degrees.

2. Place cauliflower rice into a bowl, and microwave for 5 minutes or until softened.

3. Cook beef over medium heat until it is completely brown. Then pour in the green enchilada sauce, and season with the sea salt and pepper.

4. Thoroughly mix the sour cream, onion, and cottage cheese with the cauliflower rice.

5. Place cauliflower rice mix into a casserole dish. Spread out evenly to create a layer. Then top with half of the beef mixture.

6. Add half of the shredded cheese evenly on top of the beef. Then create another layer using the remainder of the beef mixture. Add the rest of the cheddar cheese evenly on top of it.

7. Back for 20 minutes.

Macros (per serving)

Calories: 427

Fat: 29g.

Net Carbs: 6g.

Protein: 27g.

Crustless Quiche Lorraine

Servings: 4

Ingredients

- ✓ 8 Slices of bacon

- ✓ 4 Large eggs

- ✓ ¼ Tsp. sea salt

- ✓ Dash of black pepper, ground

- ✓ ¼ Tsp. nutmeg

- ✓ 1 ½ Cups heavy whipping cream

- ✓ 1 Cup Swiss cheese, shredded

- ✓ 1/3 Cup Swiss cheese, shredded

Instructions

1. Place an Instant Pot on medium sauté setting. Chop up the slices of bacon, and fry them until they're crispy. Place it aside on a paper towel.

2. Whisk together eggs in a mixing bowl. Add in whipping cream, nutmeg, sea salt, and pepper. Whisk until well blended.

3. Grease a 6 inch cake pan, and then add 1 cup of shredded Swiss cheese.

4. Crumble the cooked bacon, and add it to the cake pan.

5. Add egg batter to the cake pan.

6. Insert the steam rack into the Instant Pot, and add 1 cup of water. Lower cake pan inside of the pot, and place it on top of the steam rack. You can either cover the top of the cake pan with foil, or just wipe away the water when finished cooking.

7. Lock the lid, and cook on high pressure for 25 minutes. When done cooking, allow it to sit for 10 minutes before performing a quick pressure release.

8. Remove the cake pan, and top with the remainder of the Swiss cheese. Broil it for 5 minutes or until the cheese has a bit of brown on it.

9. Transfer the quiche onto a serving plate.

Macros (per serving)

Calories: 572

Fat: 52g.

Net Carbs: 3.5g.

Protein: 22g.

Delicious Keto Burgers

Servings: 10

Ingredients

- ✓ 28 Oz. ground turkey or beef

- ✓ 2 Tbsp. onion, finely minced

- ✓ Dash of salt

- ✓ Dash of pepper

- ✓ 4 Tbsp. cream cheese

- ✓ 2 Oz. cheddar cheese, shredded

- ✓ ¼ Tsp. garlic powder

- ✓ 1 Fresh jalapeno, diced

- ✓ 1 Tbsp. olive oil

Instructions

1. Preheat grill or broil on high. Either choice works.

2. Mix together cream cheese, cheddar cheese, garlic powder, and jalapeno in a large bowl.

3. In a separate bowl, mix together onion, salt, pepper, and meat. Divide this meat mixture into 4 separate, even pieces.

4. Flatten ¼ of the cream cheese mixture into a pancake shape. Then wrap meat around the cheese, making sure that the cheese mix is completely covered.

5. Repeat Step 4 three more times until you have used up all of the meat. Then brush each burger with a dash of olive oil.

6. Either grill or broil for about 6 minutes per side.

Macros (per serving)

Calories: 443

Fat: 34g.

Net Carbs: 4g.

Protein: 25g.

Mashed Cauliflower and Gravy

Servings: 10

Ingredients

Mashed Cauliflower

- ✓ 5 Cups chopped cauliflower

- ✓ 4 Tbsp. heavy whipping cream

- ✓ 3 Tbsp. butter

- ✓ 5 Cloves minced garlic

- ✓ 2 Tsp. rosemary

- ✓ 3 Tbsp. Parmesan

- ✓ ½ Tsp. pepper

- ✓ Dash of salt

Gravy

- ✓ 2 Cups stock or drippings

- ✓ ½ Cup heavy whipping cream

- ✓ 4 Tbsp. butter

- ✓ 1 Tsp. pepper

- ✓ ½ Tsp. xanthum gum

Instructions

Mashed Cauliflower

1. Bring a medium pot of water to a boil. There should be just enough water to cover all of the cauliflower. Add cauliflower, and boil for 15 minutes until it's tender.

2. Drain cauliflower, and place it into a food processor.

3. Add garlic, butter, and rosemary to a saucepan, and cook over medium heat until it becomes fragrant. Add to food processor, and pulse a couple of times to combine.

4. Add cream, Parmesan, salt, and pepper to the food processor until the mixture is smooth and creamy.

5. Add salt to taste.

Gravy

1. Mix together cream, broth/drippings, and butter in a saucepan, and cook on medium heat. Bring it to a boil, and then reduce heat. Simmer for 10-15 minutes.

2. Add xantum and pepper.

3. Stir continuously until gravy thickens and reduces down to your preference.

Macros (per serving)

Calories: 388

Fat: 40g.

Net Carbs: 8g.

Protein: 6g.

Mini Pizza Egg Bakes

Servings: 4

Ingredients

- ✓ 3 Large eggs, separated
- ✓ 4 Tbsp. mozzarella cheese, shredded
- ✓ 1 Tsp. Italian herb blend
- ✓ 2 Large sliced black olives
- ✓ 4 Large mild pepper rings
- ✓ 1 Tbsp. red bell pepper, diced
- ✓ 1 Tbsp. tomato sauce (make sure it has no added sugar)

Instructions

1. Sprinkle 1 Tbsp. mozzarella cheese and Italian herb seasoning into a bowl or other microwave safe dish.

2. Gently beat the egg whites so they are easier to deal with. Just don't beat them too much. You don't want them to be too frothy.

3. Pour the egg whites into each container equally. Microwave them for 90 seconds, or until they are fully cooked. Allow them to cool.

4. Lightly scramble the egg yolks.

5. Fold pizza toppings into the yolk, and then remove them from heat.

6. Top each base with ½ Tbsp. tomato sauce.

7. Add scrambled yolks and the remaining mozzarella cheese to the pizza bases. Broil in oven until the cheese is melted.

Macros (per serving)

Calories: 333

Fat: 22g.

Net Carbs: 4g.

Protein: 15g.

Roasted Leeks with Eggs

Servings: 2

Ingredients

- ✓ 2 Leeks
- ✓ 3 Green onions
- ✓ 2 Tbsp. melted ghee
- ✓ ½ Tsp. sea salt
- ✓ ¼ Tsp. black pepper, ground
- ✓ Avocado Vinaigrette
- ✓ 1 Avocado, ripe, pitted, and scooped

Instructions

1. Preheat oven to 400 degrees.

2. Cut away, and discard green tops and the bottom half-inch from leeks. Then cut them in half lengthwise.

3. Place the cut leeks and green onions onto a baking pan. Drizzle with ghee, sea salt and pepper.

4. Roast in the oven for 15 minutes or until brown.

5. Now it's time to create the vinaigrette by blending the avocado, ¾ cup olive oil, a splash of lemon juice, vinegar, salt and pepper.

6. Heat 1 tsp. olive oil in a skillet over medium heat. Cook eggs on opposite sides of the skillet until the whites just start to set, then remove leeks and onions from oven, and top them with the eggs.

7. Sprinkle red pepper and almonds onto the top of the dish. Drizzle with avocado vinaigrette.

Macros (per serving)

Calories: 204

Fat: 18g.

Net Carbs: 5g.

Protein: 6g.

Spaghetti Squash Lasagna

Servings: 10

Ingredients

- ✓ 1 Spaghetti squash

- ✓ 2 Tbsp. olive oil

- ✓ ½ Medium diced onion

- ✓ 1 Lb. breakfast sausage

- ✓ 1 Lb. ground beef

- ✓ 1 Tbsp. garlic, minced

- ✓ 24 Oz. marinara sauce (make sure it's low carb)

- ✓ 20 Oz. whole milk ricotta

- ✓ 2 Eggs, large

- ✓ ¾ Cup Parmesan cheese, grated

- ✓ 2 Tbsp. basil, chopped

- ✓ ½ Tsp. sea salt

- ✓ ½ Tsp. ground pepper

- ✓ 8 Oz. mozzarella cheese, sliced

- ✓ 2 Tbsp. parsley, chopped

Instructions

1. Preheat oven to 400 degrees.

2. Split the squash in half lengthwise and remove the seeds. Drizzle it with 1 Tbsp. olive oil, and sprinkle with salt and pepper.

3. Roast for approximately 45 minutes or until the squash is tender. It should be easy to shred with a fork. Remove from the skin, and place it to the side. Drain away any visible liquid.

4. Heat 1 Tbsp. of olive oil in a skillet. Add sausage, beef, onion, and garlic. Cook thoroughly until meat has been fully cooked. Drain away any fat/grease.

5. Add marinara sauce to the meat, and bring it to a boil. Then allow it to simmer on low for approximately 15 minutes. It should be thick.

6. Combine the ricotta and Parmesan cheese, eggs, basil, salt, and pepper in a bowl.

7. Reduce oven heat to 350 degrees and grease a casserole dish. In layers, add 1 layer of squash to the bottom of the dish. Top squash with ricotta mix. Top ricotta mix with meat sauce. Top meat sauce with a layer of mozzarella cheese.

8. Repeat adding layers as described above until you are out of mixture.

9. Sprinkle the remaining ¼ cup of Parmesan cheese and parsley on top of the lasagna.

10. Cover with foil and bake for 30 minutes. Then remove foil and bake for an additional 20 minutes. You will need to let the lasagna stand for at least 10 minutes before serving it.

Macros (per serving)

Calories: 578

Fat: 46g.

Net Carbs: 10g.

Protein: 30g.

Spinach Artichoke Chicken

Servings: 8

Ingredients

- ✓ 10 Oz. artichoke, chopped (you can use frozen or canned…check label)
- ✓ 10 Oz. chopped spinach
- ✓ 4 Oz. cream cheese
- ✓ 4 Oz. mayonnaise
- ✓ 1 Cup parmesan (separate into ½ cups)
- ✓ 1 Cup mozzarella (separate into ½ cups)
- ✓ 3 Cloves garlic
- ✓ 1 Bag chicken tenderloins

Instructions

1. Preheat oven to 400 degrees

2. Cut chicken into chunks and place them into a baking pan. Season chicken with sea salt and pepper.

3. Bake chicken for 15 minutes by itself.

4. As chicken cooks, combine spinach, artichokes, garlic, cream cheese, mayonnaise, ½ cup parmesan, and ½ cup mozzarella. Mix this extremely well.

5. When chicken has baked for 15 minutes, remove it and cover with the spinach/artichoke topping that you just created.

6. Reduce oven to 350 degrees and back chicken for 20 minutes.

7. Remove chicken from oven and sprinkle the remainder of the Parmesan and mozzarella on top of it.

8. Place oven on low broil, and place chicken back in oven until the cheese is bubbly.

Macros (per serving)

Calories: 522

Fat: 33g.

Net Carbs: 4g.

Protein: 26g.

Ultimate Breakfast Roll Ups

Servings: 5

Ingredients

- ✓ 10 Large eggs

- ✓ Dash of sea salt

- ✓ Dash of ground black pepper

- ✓ 1 ½ Cups cheddar cheese, shredded

- ✓ 5 Slices cooked bacon

- ✓ 5 Cooked breakfast sausage patties

- ✓ Nonstick cooking spray

Instructions

1. Whisk 2 eggs in a bowl, and then cook them in a skillet on medium. You should spray the skillet with nonstick spray before placing eggs into it. Season these eggs with sea salt and pepper. Cover skillet while eggs thoroughly cook.

2. Sprinkle 1/3 cup of cheese on the eggs. Lay down one strip of bacon, and then top that with sausage patty. You will then need to carefully fold the egg until it looks like a breakfast burrito.

3. Repeat this until you have 5 breakfast rolls.

Macros (per serving)

Recipes

Calories: 412

Fat: 31g.

Net Carbs: 2g.

Protein: 2

Get an Audio Book for FREE!

Don't have an Audible account?

Sign up and get "Ketogenic Diet for beginners" audio book for FREE!

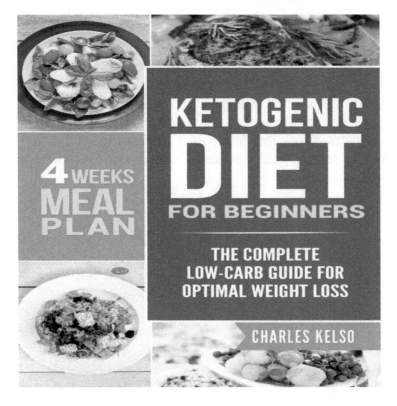

One Last Thing... Did You Enjoy the Book?

If so, then let me know by leaving a review on Amazon! Reviews are the lifeblood of independent authors. I would appreciate even a few words from you!

If you did not like the book, then please tell me! Email me at lizard.publishing@gmail.com and let me know what you didn't like. Perhaps I can change it. In today's world, a book doesn't have to be stagnant. It should be improved with time and feedback from readers like you. You can impact this book, and I welcome your feedback. Help me make this book better for everyone!

CPSIA information can be obtained
at www.ICGtesting.com
Printed in the USA
BVHW07s0102141018
530042BV00003B/3/P